ESSENTIAL OIL

FOR FIBROMYALGIA

A great home remedy

21 DIY essential oil recipes to relieve symptoms of fibromyalgia.

Beatrice .K. MacBrown

Copyright

All Rights Reserved. Contents in this book may not be copied in any way or by means without the written consent of the publisher, with the exclusion of brief excerpt in critical reviews and articles.

Beatrice .K. MacBrown© 2020

Disclaimer

This book is projected to be a general guide to raise consciousness and aid people in making knowledgeable decisions in their circumstances. This book's content is not expected to be a replacement for professional medical advice, diagnosis, or treatment.

The author takes no responsibility for any damage or injury, be it personal or monetary, due to the use or abuse of the information in this book. If you have any doubts or worries after reading this book, do well to speak to a qualified person before further actions.

Table of Content

Chapter One

What is Fibromyalgia?

Fibromyalgia (FM) or fibromyalgia syndrome (FMS) is an increasingly known protracted illness that causes pain and general discomfort in different parts of the body. The most common area of pain in the body are the body's joints, such as in the knees, hips, back, elbows, shoulders, upper chest region, and back of the head.

Fibromyalgia is an invisible illness characterized by the presence of numerous tender points and collections of symptoms.

Fibromyalgia patients may experience symptoms like

Soft tissue tenderness

Headaches and migraines

Pain, stiffness and muscle cramps

Musculoskeletal aches

Sleep disturbance and general fatigue.

Intensified sensitivity to pain

Concentration and memory

Stomach pain caused by constipation

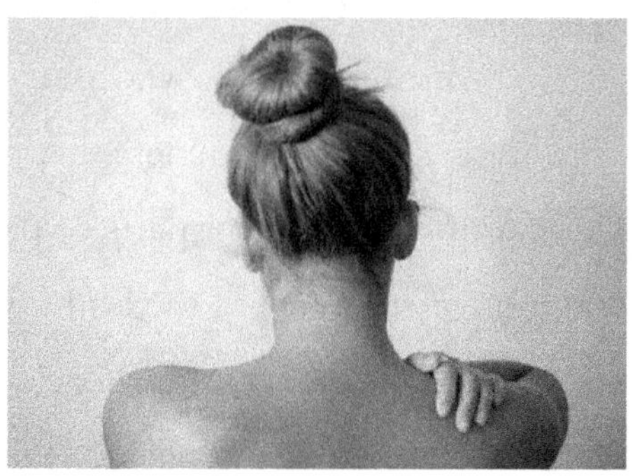

These symptoms have variable concentrations that increase and decrease over time.

According to the American College of Rheumatology, fibromyalgia affects 2–4% of people living in the United States. Fibromyalgia syndrome is not meant for particular persons though it is found more in women; that does not mean that men are ruled out. Anybody can fall victim to FM.

Presently fibromyalgia has no cure; treatment consists of dealing with the symptoms and uplifting the quality of life of the person involved.

How to diagnose fibromyalgia

According to research, there are no known laboratory tests or scan in existence for diagnosing fibromyalgia that makes it difficult for doctors to know what is causing the pains and aches.

The rheumatologist (Doctor) will ask you about your health and family history and rely on them. After getting the self-reported symptoms, the doctor will proceed with a proper physical examination and an accurate manual tender point examination. The examination performed by the doctor is based on the standardized ACR criteria.

After the examination, your doctor will want to rule out any other problems by first taking your blood sample to check hormone levels or possibly look for signs of inflammation. Secondly, you may require to get an X-rays so she/he can take a look at your bones.

Fibromyalgia is not a one-time diagnosis. It takes an average of five years to have the condition diagnosed.

What causes fibromyalgia?

Presently no one can pinpoint what causes fibromyalgia, but new research points to a disorder involving neurotransmitter/neuroendocrine dysregulation. The pains seem to increases because of the abnormal sensory processing in the central nervous system. FM patients suffer numerous physiological abnormalities. These include a decrease in levels of blood flow to the thalamus region of the brain, high levels of substance P inside the spinal cord, decreased serotonin and tryptophan, and HPA axis hypofunction and abnormalities in cytokine function.

What causes Fibromyalgia outburst?

Emotional stress and traumatic injuries that may cause Fibromyalgia outburst are:

Past surgical operations

Accidents that lead to injuries

First pregnancy and childbirth

Emotional stress such as separation in marriage or death of a family member or a friend

Fibromyalgia Symptoms

Some people suffering from FM experience high sensitive to medicines and may choose to use more natural health care options.

Coping with the persistent pain and exhaustion of fibromyalgia can be quite demanding. To relieve the stress is to find a way to reduce the overall symptom of this protracted illness. Fibromyalgia involves abnormalities in neurological sensitivity. Therefore soothing physically and emotionally practices most times bring a sense of relief. According to research, aromatherapy alone or also with massage and other relaxation methods can help reduce the symptoms. Essential oil is an aromatic material with a beautiful and powerful fragrant used for health care practices.

The use of essential oils can help calm the mind, promote sleep, increase circulation, reduce muscle pain, relieve headaches and enhance the overall well-being. The essential oil provides momentary relief from chronic pain

Chapter Two

Essential oils for Fibromyalgia Pain

The natural healing properties and health benefits of essential oil are great home remedies for fibromyalgia patients. They have therapeutic potential for pain management, offering relief from the physical and mental symptoms of fibromyalgia. Mental symptoms can be depression and anxiety.

Essential oils must be diluted with a carrier oil before applying to the skin to avoid allergic reactions or irritation. You can also use essential oil as an aromatherapy technique by diffusing it in the air or inhaling.

Always discuss with your doctor before using essential oil for fibromyalgia.

NOTE: You are advised to use at least 6 teaspoons of carrier oil for every 15 drops of essential oil

Common Carrier oils for dilutions are:

Dilute few drops of essential oil with 1 ounce (2 tablespoons) of carrier oil

Grape seed oil

Almond oil

Massage oil

Olive oil

Coconut oil (fractionated)

Avocado oil

Unscented lotions

For therapeutic massage purposes, use up to 10 or 12 drops of a blend of essences in a 1-ounce base of carrier oil.

Essential oils can be used in many ways:

1. Pain Relief: Apply diluted essential oils to the skin by massaging or physical therapy. The diluted oil is absorbed little by little into the skin as the massaging is going on. It helps to reduce inflammation and fibromyalgia pain.

2. Aromatherapy: This is the process by which essential oil is aerated or diffused in the air for inhaling of their scent. When inhaled, it reduces

the effect of migraines, stress, pain, anxiety, and insomnia.

3. Soothing: Through the hot bath process, pain relief and aromatherapy is combined. The technique is called soothing. During the hot bath, warm water enhances blood circulation, which helps reduces pain. The essential oils added to the bath penetrate the skin, thereby blocking pain. The steam that is coming from the bathtub also forms aromatherapy.

Natural essential oils are quite useful in calming various symptoms of fibromyalgia.

Nevertheless, there are some guidelines you must follow before using essential oil for fibromyalgia.

- o   Essential oils are highly concentrated and toxic; please do not consume.
- o   If you observe that you are allergic or sensitive to any of them, discontinue its use immediately.
- o   Make sure you purchase a high-quality essential oil
- o   Look out for side effect after each use

The most useful essential oils in treating some of the
FM symptoms are:

- Lavender Oil

Lavender is one of the natural essential oils that treat
fibromyalgia's two main symptoms: pain and anxiety.
Lavender helps in alleviating the pain fibromyalgia
brings. Many people who have fibromyalgia find it
difficult to sleep at night.

The Lavender aromatic and stress-relieving properties
help increase blood circulation in patients bringing
about more comfortable sleep, reduce inflammation and
soothe fatigued nerve.

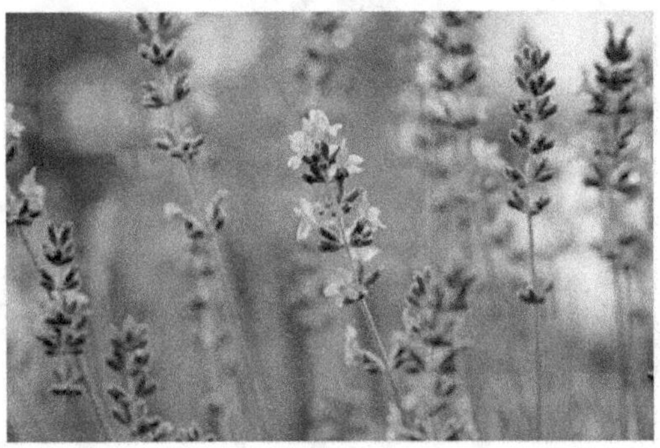

Lavender essential oil also helps to soothe other
fibromyalgia associated symptoms like headaches,
nausea, migraines and depression.

- Peppermint Oil

Peppermint oil is an ideal essential oil for people living with fibromyalgia. One of the problems experienced by people living with fibromyalgia is the inability to concentrate appropriately, often called fibro fog or brain fog. Peppermint oil has anti-inflammatory and anti-spasmodic properties that help reduce pain, muscle spasms or cramps, clear brain fog and fatigue.

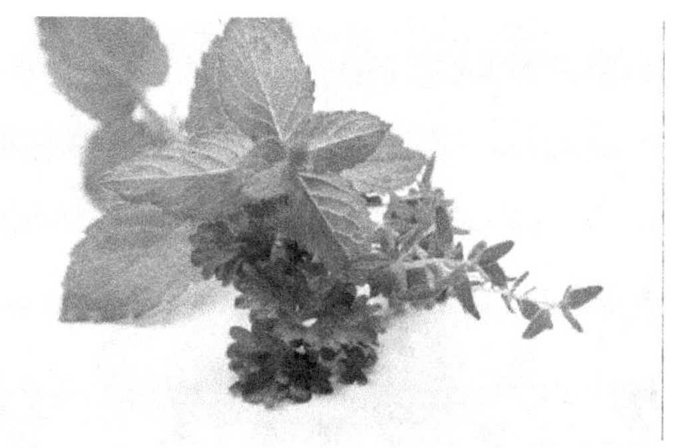

It also counters the effect of other fibromyalgia symptoms. Peppermint essential oil has other health benefits, including boosting nervous system health, reducing congestion, and improving memory.

- Capsaicin Oil

Capsaicin is among the best essential oil for fibromyalgia. It is derived from red chili peppers, and it is known as a pain reliever. It has an anti-inflammatory property that, when applied directly to the area of pain, gives temporary pain relief to patients. Capsaicin oil can also alleviate pain caused by osteoarthritis.

- Cedarwood Oil

Cedarwood essential oil for fibromyalgia is gotten from the cedarwood plant. When inhaled, its property relieves pain by bringing into life a pathway of the brain that deals with pain. It also has a calming effect on the body.

- Ginger and Citrus Oils

Ginger and citrus make up an excellent combination of essential oils for fibromyalgia. Their aromatic property helps in relieving stress. When ginger and citrus fruit are used as an aromatherapy treatment, they help in relieving acute bone fracture pain and other treatment according to study.

Ginger and citrus essential oils aromatherapy treatment provide some benefits for fibromyalgia patients when used alongside other treatments.

- Ginger Oil

Ginger is a known essential oil for reducing nausea and improves digestion. Many people living with fibromyalgia suffer from nausea and dizziness. Ginger oil has a lot of health benefits, including lowering inflammation and blocked pain sensations and reducing muscle pain. It also increases antioxidant activity in the body.

- Basil Oil

Apart from cooking basil essential oil has other health benefits.

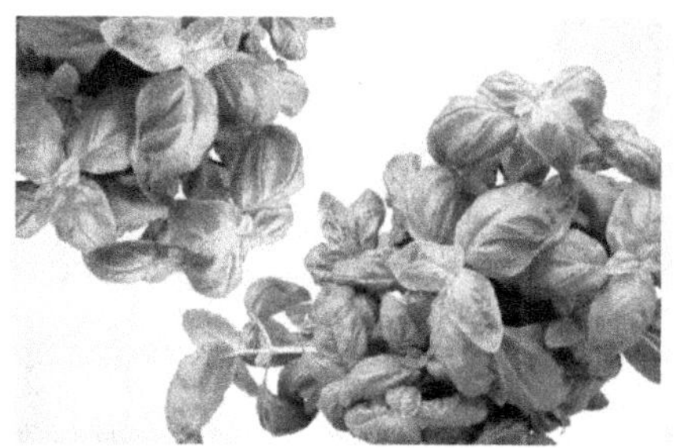

Basil oil is an effective pain relief remedy for fibromyalgia patients. It reduces swelling and inflammation in fibromyalgia patients when used correctly. Basil essential oil also eases nausea, headaches, mental clarity and strength. It treats nervous tension, melancholy, fatigue and depression when used as aromatherapy.

- Helichrysum oil

Helichrysum oil is one of the most popular essential oil for fibromyalgia pain. The oil is derived from the flower of a plant by steam distilling process. The word "helichrysum is a Greek word. It has anti-oxidant and anti-inflammation properties that reduce muscular pains, tension, reduces swelling and inflammation. It also improves blood circulation in the body.

- Black pepper

Black pepper essential oil is hot and spicy, which gives it the power to the relieve pain felt in the muscles and joints It helps reduce pain, keep the muscles warm, and improve circulation, ease stiffness of the joints and fatigue. Black pepper oil is a potent oil and should use sparingly with caution.

- Juniper

Juniper is an essential oil that is highly recommended for people living with fibromyalgia.

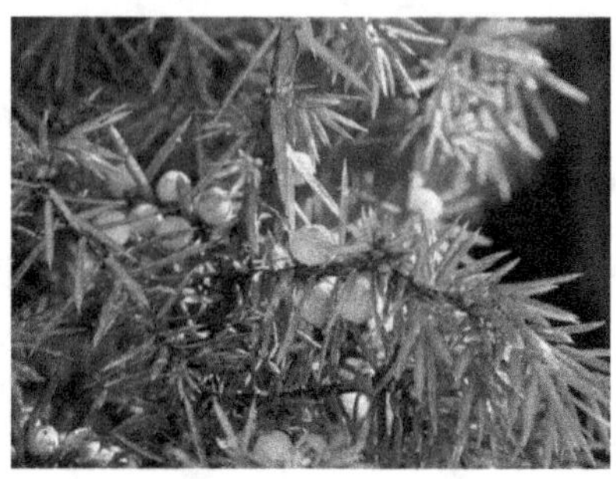

When applied topically, the oil helps stimulate the mind, reduces muscle spasms, and joints/muscle pain. It also has a very relaxing quality and a super nerve-calming quality.

- Eucalyptus

Eucalyptus oil is extracted from a powerful tree known as Eucalyptus. The oil has anti-inflammatory and decongestant properties. Eucalyptus is best for blood circulation and supply, and it plays a vital role in flushing out toxins from the body. According to a study carried on people with a total knee replacement, the oil can also be used to reduce muscle aches, lower pain and inflammation, and soreness.

- **Sandalwood oil**

Sandalwood oil is extracted from the aromatic sandalwood tree. The oil is known for its antiseptic and anti-inflammatory effects. Sandalwood oil contains a substance called santalol, which has depressant and soothing effects on the central nervous system. When Sandalwood oil is inhale, it can calm, sedate, improve sleep and increase non-rapid eye movement. Sandalwood oil also possesses a lingering soothing odour that helpsrelieve tension, depression and confusion, which come with people suffering from chronic pain.

- Roman chamomile

Roman chamomile is term great all-purpose essential oil. It is an excellent oil for stress relief and relaxation. Roman chamomile is good at calming the mind and body during severe fibromyalgia attack to stay positive. The oil can be useful in relieving fibromyalgia symptoms because it is a nerve sedative and has anti-spasmodic properties. It helps people who have fibromyalgia to overcome their difficulty to sleep by improving sleep.

- Jasmine

Jasmine essential oil is another alternative for those suffering from sleep-deprived symptoms of fibromyalgia. It has a sedative nature to help people find more peaceful sleep. Jasmine oil also has antispasmodic and some anti-depressant qualities for those suffering from restless leg syndrome, and it is soothing.

- Marjoram

Marjoram essential oil is extracted from the leaves of marjoram plants by a steam distillation process. The oil may help reduce headache pain, reduce stress, anxiety and provide a more peaceful sleep. Occasionally you need to mix it with other essential oil to help fight pain and insomnia.

- Rose

A rose is a beautiful flower, and the smell is fantastic. Rose essential oil derives from rose tree help promotes sleep by reducing insomnia. It is also refreshing and has the ability to relieve pain.

- Neroli

Neroli oil is highly recommended for reducing fibromyalgia anxiety and stress. Neroli oil is a combination of slight citrus and floral aromas. It's been suggested that neroli oil can reduce inflammation, muscle spasms, stress, cortisol levels, and blood pressure associated with fibromyalgia.

Neroli is the right essential oil for memory improvement and other cognitive issues.

- Clary sage

Clary sage has anticonvulsant, antidepressant, antispasmodic, astringent, and antiseptic properties. It is an excellent and highly-recommended essential oil for fibromyalgia patients. Clary sage plays a vital role in improving mood, soothing anxiety, and reducing depression in people living with fibromyalgia pain.

- Rosemary

People who suffer fibro fog should make rosemary essential oil their friend. According to a study, rosemary oil improves memory by boosting nerve growth factor. This process eases fibro fog symptoms. It also supports the healing of neurological tissue, brain functioning, relieves muscle aches, and soothe nausea.

- Cypress

Cypress oils are great option to reduce fatigue and stress. It possesses an antispasmodic property, which is a real benefit. Cypress oil works well in reducing menstrual cramps and hot flashes associated with women's fibromyalgia sufferer.

- Melissa

Melissa oil is a rare oil used to calm inflammation and reduce the feeling of depression. It also helps improve nervous system disorder and the health of the immune system.

- Bergamot

Bergamot essential oil is an excellent natural option for fibromyalgia pain. It is slightly sweet and slightly floral, a combination of neroli and lavender.

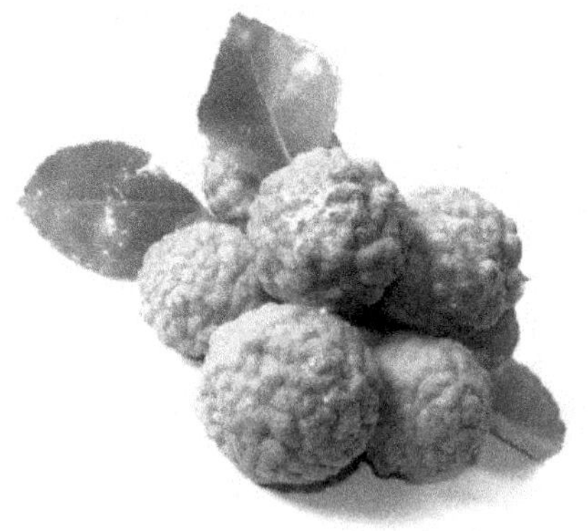

The oil has been in existence for treating stress, nerve pain, tension, and help for people down with depression.

- Grapefruit

Grapefruit essential oil has stimulating effects on the mind and body. When the oil stimulates the brain, it makes the brain active by giving it a new direction of thinking. It keeps the body's metabolism in proper order by stimulating the endocrinal glands and promoting adequate secretion of enzymes and hormones. It also stimulates the nervous system making people more alert and active.

- Ylang Ylang

Ylang-Ylang essential oil is extracted from the fresh flower of the Cananga tree. It contains analgesic and pain-relieving properties. These properties offer excellent relief for fibromyalgia patients.

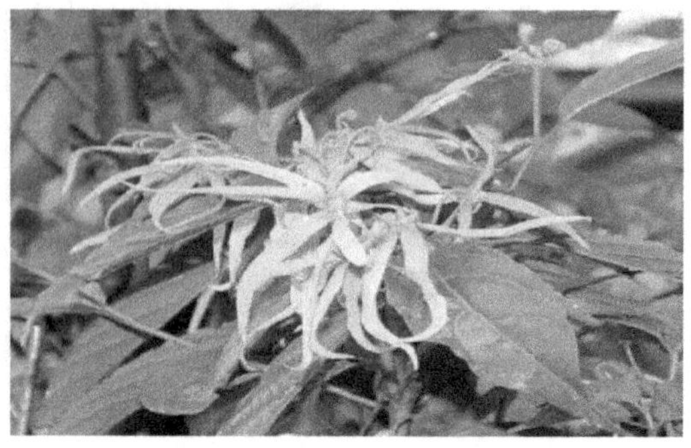

Ylang-ylang oil helps in treating high blood pressure and promotes rest

- Vetiver

Vetiver oil has been used for thousands of years in traditional medicine in Asia and West Africa. The oil is excellent in improving energy levels, soothing anxiety, and cooling of the body.

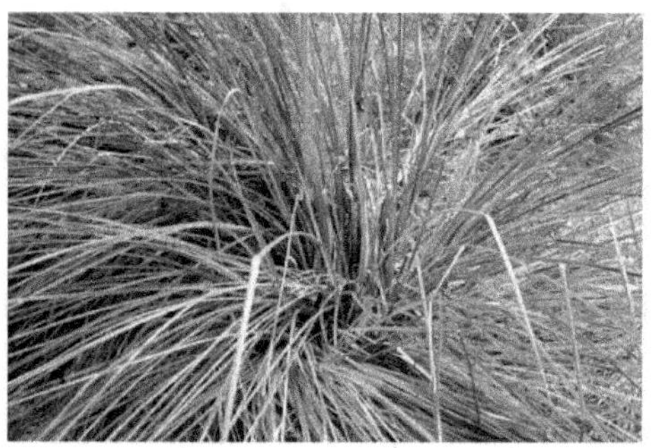

Chapter Three

Essential oil recipes for fibromyalgia

1.   Relaxing massage recipe

Regular massage can help reduce chronic pain experienced while living with fibromyalgia. The massage therapy help to improve sleeping patterns, reduced stress hormones and raises serotonin levels.

Ingredients:

4 oz amber glass jar

1/4cup or 4 tablespoons of coconut oil (carrier oil)

1/4 cup or 4 tablespoons of shea oil

10 drops of lemongrass oil

5 drops of vetiver oil

5 drops of ginger oil

Method

Put a heat-safe bowl carefully on top of a pot of boiling water over medium-low heat, melt the coconut oil and shea butter until it is in liquid form. Allow to cool for some minutes, say 2-3 minutes.

Add the essential oils in the carrier oils

Mix until well blended and store in an amber bottle.

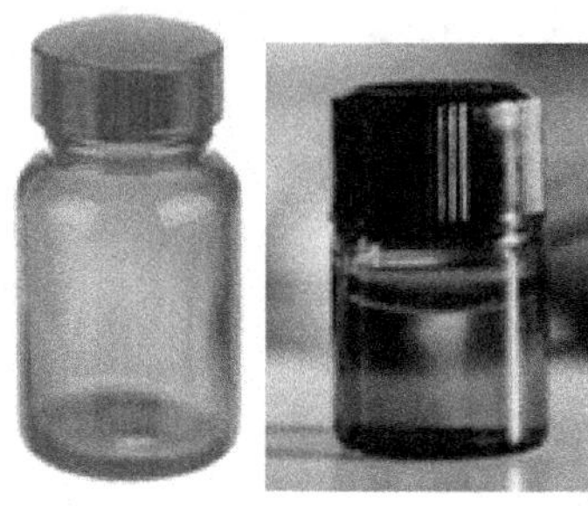
Amber bottle

Use for massage on the affected area.

2. Healing bath recipe

Taking baths is an age-long pain reliever practice for people suffering from fibromyalgia consistent soreness. The heat that comes from water loosens stiff muscles and gives body comfort. Especially if it is loaded with essential oils

Ingredients:

1 cup of Epsom salts

20 drops of spearmint oil

20 drops of geranium oil

10 drops of chamomile oil

Method:

Bring a clean bowl; pour Epsom salt inside the bowl. Then add the essentials oils one after the other. Mix and pour the mixture inside the bath. The essential oils and Epsom salts will give you the relief you desire.

Soak your body for 15 – 30 minutes in the bath to reap the essential oils' benefits.

3. Sustainable relief bath recipe

The blend is a quick one that can be found in your kitchen cabinet.

Ingredients:

5 drops black pepper oil

15 drops of rosemary oil

6 drops of marjoram

Methods

Measure the blend and add it to your bathwater. Soak your body inside the bathe for 15 to 20 minutes. The spicy blend helps to relieve the pain for some time and gives you a soothing sleep.

4. Fibromyalgia buster recipe

This is a quick recipe to prepare and carry around. Apply anytime you experience an increase in pain in your pressure points. It helps to relieve pain when applied periodically throughout the day.

Ingredients:

10 ml Roller bottle

20 drops of chamomile oil

20 drops of lavender oil

20 drops of wild orange oil

20 drops of marjoram oil

1/2 cup of coconut oil (fractionated)

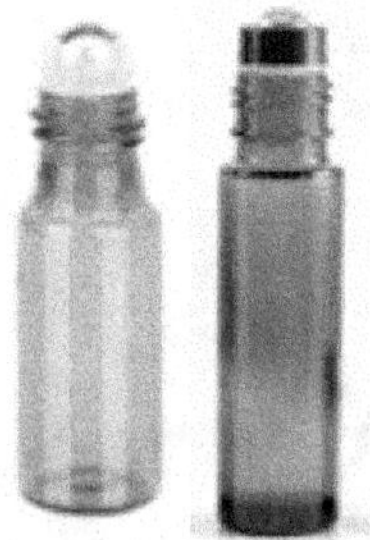 Roller bottle

Method

Pour all of the essential oils in the roller bottle with a funnel and fill the remaining space with the coconut oil.

Before you use, roll the bottle between your hands for sometimes to ensure that the carrier and essential oils are properly mix.

Shake thoroughly by rolling the bottle between your hands for 30 seconds before use. This is to ensure that the essential oil and carrier oil are well blended.

5. Roller recipe

Ingredients:

2 drops of lavender oil

2 drops of vetiver oil

2 drops of marjoram oil

2 drops of chamomile oil

2 drops of geranium oil

1 drop of frankincense oil

1 drop of ginger oil

1 ounce or 2 tablespoons carrier oil

Method

Mix well and store it in a roller bottle. Apply to the affected area.

6. pain relief recipe 1

Ingredients

4 oz of an amber bottle

4 drops of Ginger

4 drops Black pepper

2 drops of Clary sage

4 drops of Clove

1 ounce of Avocado (carrier oil)

Method

Put a heat-safe bowl carefully on top of a pot of boiling water over medium-low heat, melt the coconut oil until it is in liquid form. Allow to cool for some minutes, say 2-3 minutes.

Add the essential oils in the carrier oil

Mix until well blended and store in an amber bottle.

Use to massage the affected area.

7. Pain relief recipes 2

The essential oils for this recipe are handy and easy to get for aromatherapy fans.

Ingredients:

4 oz amber bottle

1 ounce or 2 tablespoons of carrier oil

2 drops of peppermint oil

2 drops of clove oil

3 drops of frankincense oil

1 drop of eucalyptus oil

Method

Mix the ingredients and store them in a dark amber bottle. It can be added during bathing for immediate relief.

8. Balm recipes for pain

The recipe is almost the same with the lotion but with a little thickness.

Ingredients:

2 drops of ginger oil

3 drops of clove oil

5 drops of eucalyptus oil

5 drops of peppermint oil

1 tablespoon avocado oil

1/2 teaspoons of vitamin E

2 ounces of virgin coconut oil

1 oz Beeswax

Methods

Put a heat-safe bowl carefully on top of a pot of boiling water over medium-low heat; melt the coconut oil and beeswax until they are in liquid form. Allow to cool for some minutes, say 2-3 minutes. Add vitamin E

Add the essential oils in the carrier oil and mix thoroughly.

Pour inside the amber bottle with a funnel.

Apply to the affected area and keep out of reach of children.

9. Anti-inflammatory synergy recipe

The mixture of these essential oils will help to relax muscle tension and reduce swelling.

Ingredients

5 drops of Lavender

5 drops of Helichrysum

3 drops of Peppermint

1 oz of Avocado oil (carrier oil)

Method

Add the essential oils in the carrier oil

Mix until well blended and store in an amber bottle.

Use to massage the affected area.

10. Tension and swelling recipe

This blend relaxes muscle spasms, tension and soothes inflammation

Ingredients:

1 ounce or 2 tablespoons of Olive oil (carrier oil)

2 drops of Cypress oil

2 drops of Sandalwood oil

Method

Pour the ingredients in the amber bottle and mix thoroughly. Apply directly to the affected area where the pain is high. Keep all oil away from the eyes.

11. Swelling relief only

Combination of these oil help to relieve inflammation swelling or bruising.

Ingredients

4 oz glass jar

5 drops of Arnica oil.

5 drops of Lemongrass oil.

1 ounce or 2 tablespoons of carrier oil of your choice.

Method

Mix the ingredients and pour them inside an amber bottle.

Apply directly to the affected area for ease relief of pains from an illness.

12. Spray for Calming Sleep

Some of the symptoms most fibromyalgia patients suffer from are sleep disturbances and insomnia. But it can be taken care of with the blend of these essential oils.

Ingredients

4 tablespoons of rubbing alcohol

4 tablespoon of distilled water

10 drops of lavender essential oil

10 drops of sandalwood oil

10 drops of marjoram oil

4 ounces amber glass spray bottle

Method

Pour the ingredients carefully in a glass spray bottle with a stainless steel funnel, cover the lid, and shake thoroughly to combine.

Spray the blend on the bed sheet and pillowcase before sleep.

13. Stress/anxiety relief recipe:

Ingredients

1 ounce or 2 tablespoons of carrier oil

12 drops of any of the below listed essential oils

Rose otto essential oil

Clary sage oil

Frankincense oil

Sweet orange oil

Bergamot oil

ylang ylang oil

Grapefruit oil

Sandalwood oil

Sweet marjoram

Neroli oil

Petitgrain oil

Mandarin oil

Rose geranium oil

Tangerine

Lavender oil

Jasmine oil

Method

Pour any of the listed essential oil of your choice with a carrier oil in a diffuser. Place on a table or hang in your room or a convenient place. Inhale as it diffuses.

14. Peaceful sleep recipe:

Add the blend in your diffuser for a peaceful sleep.

The mixture reduces joint pains.

Ingredients:

2 drop of valerian oil

2 drop of lavender oil

4 drops of mandarin oil

Method

In a diffuser pour water and add the listed oil.

15. Harmony and safety feeling recipes:

Ingredients

2 oz. diffuser bottle or bigger

2 drops of Frankincense

2 drops of Lavender

1 drop of Rose

1 drop of Mandarin

1 drop of Neroli

I drop helichrysum.

2 oz carrier oil

Method

Pour any of the listed essential oil and carrier oil in a diffuser. Place on a table or hang in your room or a convenient place. Inhale as it diffuses.

16. headaches recipe:

Ingredients

4 oz amber bottle

4 drops of Lavender oil

6 drops of Peppermint oil

2 drops of Marjoram oil

2 drops of Roman chamomile

1 oz of carrier oil

Pour the listed essential oil and carrier oil in a diffuser. Place on a table or hang in your room or a convenient place. Inhale as it diffuses.

17. Increased circulation recipe 1:

Ingredients

4 oz amber bottle

2 drops of Rosemary oil

4 drops of Ginger oil

1 drop of Black pepper

1 drop of Peppermint

1 drop of Lemongrass

4 drops of Rose geranium

1 oz of carrier oil

Method

Mix all the ingredients and pour them with funnel a in an amber bottle. Store in a dark place and use it for massage.

18. Increase circulation recipe 2

Ingredients

4 drops of lavender oil

1 drop of frankincense oil

4 drops of sweet orange oil

1 drop of neroli oil

Method

Mix all the ingredients and pour them with a funnel in an amber bottle. Store in a dark place and use it for massage.

Increase circulation recipe 3

Ingredients

8 drops of sweet marjoram

2 drop of Roman chamomile

8 drops of mandarin

2 drop of rose

Method

Mix all the ingredients and pour them with a funnel in an amber bottle. Store in a dark place and use it for massage.

19. Increase circulation recipe 4

Ingredients

4 drops of lavender

4 drops of rose geranium

2 drops of rosemary

1 drop of lemongrass

Method

Mix all the ingredients and pour them with a funnel in an amber bottle. Store in a dark place and use it for massage.

Experiment the above-listed blend for an increase in circulation and use the on that works best for you.

20. Fibro compress

For some time now, compress has been used as a remedy for pain relief. A compress is a cloth soaked in warm or cold water firmly pressed to the sea of pain.

Ingredients:

1 teaspoon of rosemary oil

50 drops of lavender oil

50 drops of marjoram oil

1 oz of carrier oil of your choice

Method

In a clean bowl, combine the ingredients. Mix thoroughly and add a cup of hot water. Get a cloth, soak it inside the mixture, and apply it to the affected area. To keep the cloth together secure with plastic wrap. Use regularly to keep the pain away.

21. DIY general fibromyalgia massage recipe

This method is amazing because it penetrates the pain giving you relieve you so much desire. The mixture is useful in tackling the pain in the joints and muscles. Use regularly to reduce the pain say every four hours.

Ingredients

3 ounces of Mama Z's Oil Base

2 drops of Bergamot Oil

2 drops of Camphor Oil

2 drops of Lemon Oil

2 drops of Peppermint Oil

2 drops of Rosemary Oil

4 oz Glass Jar

Method

In a clean bowl, pour Mama Z's oil, mix thoroughly with a spatula until well blended.

Pour the mixture in an amber glass jar and store in the refrigerator. Shake and apply on the affected area every four hours.

Conclusion

Risks and considerations involving essential oil

Essential oils are great natural remedies, but they are also some risk attached to it.

The following are some precautions to be taken if you want to use essential oil for a natural remedy.

Do not ingest essential oils; they are highly concentrated and have a serious side effect if taken orally.

Make sure you test essential oil before use to avoid an allergic reaction. To check, mix your choice essential oil with carrier oil and test on the forearm.

Check for unnecessary side effects. If you notice any side effect, discontinues use immediately and consults your doctor. Side effects vary from an individual concerning age, health, and drugs.

Make sure you dilute the essential oil with a carrier oil to avoid skin irritation, rashes, or blistering.

Make sure your essential oil is of good quality; get from a reputable brand.